# Sexuality and Addiction